Contents

Introduction:

Chapter 1: Time restricted eating and why you should avoid intermittent fasting.......7

Chapter 2: How we burn fat and therapeutic fasting.......24

Chapter 3: The 48-hour fast: Accelerating fat loss and cell repair.......40

Chapter 4: The 72-hour fast: Unlocking your body's ability to heal itself.......54

Chapter 5: The only 5-day fast I would recommend.......58

Chapter 6: Spirituality and closing.......63

Introduction

As I sit here compiling this book, I'm currently on hour 19 of my fast. My client, Vanessa, is probably on hour 32 or so. We often check up on each other to make sure that we're navigating our fasts safely and effectively. Fasting is as much a battle of the mind as it is of the body, but the results are undeniable.

Now, the goals Vanessa and I have for our fasts are very different. My main goal is to reclaim the lifestyle that I once had before I was diagnosed with primary-progressive multiple sclerosis. Basically, I don't want to walk with a cane for the rest of my life; and I can't even fathom the thought of the disease progressing further. Vanessa's primary goal, on the other hand, has always been fat loss and body toning, but she has also been able to improve some gastrointestinal issues that have bothered her for years. And we both are using the same simple, effective secret weapon to achieve our goals: *water fasting*.

I have a lot to say about water fasting, but let me first tell you a little more about my background. Back in 2010 I started a gym called BFF Boot Camp. My goal was to create a results-driven fitness program that would allow people to attain the personal goals they walk in with, which are usually fat loss and toning. The biggest challenge that most people have when it comes to changing their bodies and improving their health is the nutrition aspect, so I've made my best effort to give people easy tools to get to their end-goal as quickly and safely as possible.

Around 2015, I started to notice that my own body was acting erratically. At first, I brushed it off as a bad day at the gym, and then I started to notice loss of coordination. Within 18 months, I found myself being wheeled to the hospital in a wheelchair to receive massive steroid injections for what would later be diagnosed as an aggressive form of multiple sclerosis.

Even after my diagnosis, I continued training my clients and remained committed to helping them achieve their end-goals. However, I also dedicated myself to finding alternatives to injections as treatment for my disease. The main objection that I had to my neurologists was that they didn't offer any kind of daily actionable habit that I could implement in order to slow down the progression of the disease. Instead, they always leaned toward prescribing pharmaceutical drugs. And while I am grateful for the creation of these drugs to diminish symptoms or slow down progression of the disease, it appeared that none of them were going to be effective in reversing my condition, which was, of course, what I most wanted to happen.

So, after looking through countless articles and videos of people who had achieved success in reversing chronic diseases, I came across the idea of water fasting. After reading up on it, I decided to implement this technique myself.

Now, I'm going to be honest with you: Being diagnosed with an "incurable" progressive disease that is expected to take away the things you enjoy most in life tends to have an effect on your whole person—mentally, physically, and emotionally. Because of the toll my illness was having on me, I wasn't able to work out as often as I wanted, and I often battled depression and ate in a way that wasn't always consistent with my profession. As a result, not surprisingly, I gained more than a few extra pounds. Before long, I grew ashamed of my body and hid behind baggy clothes, hoping to somehow find my way back to the identity I had previously enjoyed for 34 years.

That's where I was when I decided to implement water fasting. And to my surprise, at the end of my first fast, I noticed something that I had not seen for a while: abs! But I wasn't the only one who noticed. Everybody—my clients included—would come up to me and ask how much weight I had lost. At first, I was reluctant to tell them that I had been water fasting, because I didn't know enough about it to advise on the matter. There has been so much literature out there that says if you don't have three square meals a day, with three snacks in between, you're going to lose muscle, you're going to make your bones brittle, and you're ultimately going to put yourself in the hospital. So, I wasn't yet willing to go against that advice. But as I continued using water fasting, I started to notice other fringe benefits, including increased energy levels. And when I did exercise, my performance improved for a period of time after the fast.

So, water fasting became a regular habit for me. And because there were times during the fast when I would become cranky, I began warning my clients ahead of time that I was about to start a water fast and to please just excuse me if I wasn't quite myself. Bear in mind that I taught classes starting at five in the morning, so I usually had to wake up at around 4:15. Going that long of a day while on a water fast and having to be physically active, yelling, thinking, and communicating with clients—that can all take a toll on you. So, I asked my clients to please forgive me if I didn't seem myself, and I would let them know when it was over.

The one thing that my clients would not leave me alone about was the fact that I would be thinner after each fast, and they wanted the results that I was getting. So, I decided to dig deeper and see if there was any literature out there that might suggest that water fasting could actually be safe for these clients. And, lo and behold, I found it. After that, once I was able to feel comfortable giving advice on fasting, I decided to help people along with the process.

Please understand, though, that getting used to fasting takes time. I often tell people that if you jump into the deep end of the water fasting "pool" without proper preparation, you're probably going to hate me, your life, and all your surroundings! True, a longer fast yields more results than a shorter one. But you can do some real damage to your social life if you aren't prepared for the effects. So, in addition to the physical, chemical, and physiological effects of water fasting, there are important practical and psychological aspects to consider. This is important to remember if you want to fast correctly, without assaulting your co-workers or losing your temper with your family.

Before we go any further, then let me emphasize that water fasting is going to be a process. It is very simple, and it 100% works. But it's not all that easy on the mind. It's going to take some time to get yourself to a point where you can fast without becoming everybody's worst nightmare. But if your goals include fat loss, toning, improving your metabolism, and increasing your energy, you can reasonably expect get that with water fasting. And if your goals go even beyond that, perhaps this information can open your world to the full powers of fasting.

Now, keep in mind, the advice I'll give you in this book is not meant to replace the advice of your primary care provider. Anytime you begin any kind of health or diet modification program, you should run it past your primary care physician first. Although I am convinced that what I share here can be of real benefit to you, this is, ultimately, the chronicle of my own journey into water fasting and how it has transformed my life. It's a story that I'm eager to share it with you.

Chapter One

Time-Restricted Eating and Why You Should *Avoid* Intermittent Fasting

I realize that the introduction may have gotten you excited, and you can't wait to start water fasting; however, as I mentioned, it's important to understand that there is a process involved in water-fasting effectively. If you're highly motivated and looking for a quick fix, you might be inclined to jump into fasting immediately, but odds are you'll end up miserable, and therefore make the people around you miserable. Moreover, if you continue to exercise poor nutritional habits between, and immediately following, your water fasts, it won't be long before you see negative results. In addition, as you progress into longer-term water fasting, you're going to have to learn how to break your water fast effectively so as to not shock your digestive system. With all this in mind, then, we're going to take a step back and first get you to a point where your body is ready for a water fast without shocking it.

That's where time-restricted eating comes in. The more commonly used term for this is intermittent fasting. But the terms are interchangeable. Essentially, you limit the amount of hours in day that you eat. Most people don't understand this concept, so we're going to spend some time covering it in this chapter. The good news is that time-restricted eating is a very effective way of preparing your body for your very first, short-term water fasts.

Now, before we get into this, understand that I've been training clients for 20 years, and I've run my own fat-loss-focused boot camp since 2010. So, I have dealt with literally thousands of men and women who want to lose weight and tone up, and they always tell me the same thing: They want to firm up their midsection and perhaps get rid of their "bat wings" (the fat underneath their arms), and they're willing to do anything to accomplish that.

The first thing I usually do is arrange a consultation with them to find out what they're putting into their bodies and what their lifestyles are like. At these consultations I often hear that they're encountering the exact same lifestyle pitfalls: they're not getting enough sleep, they're definitely not getting enough water, and they're overly stressed out. And then when we discuss their intake of food, it's clear that they have a warped idea of what it takes to lose weight.

But it's not really their fault, because the media does such a great job in getting people to believe that fat is bad, that carbohydrates are bad, that you should be eating primarily protein, and that you need to cut your daily calories to 1200 or less. And if you do all this over time, you're told that you'll successfully lose weight. Understandably, though, people struggle with this regimen.

Another reason they struggle is that even though they're taking in 1200 calories or less, they're stretching those calories out over an extremely long eating period. So, they've been conditioned to have six to seven meals a day on a total of just 1200 calories, which means they're giving their bodies these short bursts of caloric intake. And this stressful regimen usually ends up including one or two "meals" of the worst combination of caloric intake that you can consume: the combination of fat and sugar. So, when you consider the combined effects of all of these habits that people are practicing every day, it's going to be very hard for them to see success. In fact, this might describe you.

The first thing that I had to address in order to help my clients, then, was the metabolic and physiological effects of eating so many times throughout the course of a day. I looked around on the internet to see if I could find a resource that would allow people to see the error in their ways, and I came across a very reputable doctor named Rhonda Patrick, who explained the concept of time-restricted eating. Based on what this doctor said, one of the first things that I began telling people to do was to restrict their "eating window"—the time between their first meal and their last meal—to no more than 12 hours.

And here's why: When you wake up in the morning and you consume anything that's not water—including tea, coffee, or your favorite bagel—it starts all these metabolic processes within your system, including in your gut and liver. Essentially, all of these processes operate on a clock, because we are not nocturnal creatures, we're diurnal, which basically means that we're awake when the sun is out and we're built to be asleep when it's dark outside. So, a lot of these processes are kicked off with the exposure to light and the consumption of food. And this kickoff process lasts about 12 hours, because that's how the body is essentially geared to work. When you continue eating beyond those 12 hours, your body's metabolism of the food you eat becomes inefficient.

So, I brought this concept over to the clients in my gym and suggested that they make it a goal to eat only within a 12-hour window. If, for example, their first meal was at 7 a.m., then their last meal would be at 7 p.m. If their first meal was at 10 a.m., their last meal could be as late as 10 p.m. The one other piece of advice I offered was that, to the best of their ability, they should avoid consuming anything other than water the last three hours before they went to sleep, as this might help with digestion. To somebody who was really struggling with that idea I would say, "At the very least, try to make sure that whatever you consume those last three hours before you go to bed is liquid only."

It turned out that a lot of my clients struggled to keep all of their eating within a 12-hour period. Many of my clients were moms, and many moms really don't start their day until their kids are asleep. So, first thing in the morning they get their kids ready for school, and they may munch on something while they're preparing the kids' lunches. After that, they may not eat much at all until that evening after the kids are asleep. At that point, maybe while they're doing the laundry, they'll snack on something while they watch TV.

In many such cases, then, what should have been a 12-hour window for eating was actually a 16-, 17-, or even 18-hour window. To make matters worse, many of these same moms also struggled with sleep. So, even though they were consuming relatively few calories throughout the day and evening, by eating across such a wide window of time, they were becoming less insulin sensitive, which caused them to begin wasting muscle. Ironically, then, the very thing that a lot of people worry about when they think of fasting is actually being done to them by the very large feeding windows in their current lifestyle.

There was a study done on time-restricted eating in rats by Dr. Satchin Panda out of the Salk Institute. What he found was that if the mice were to eat beyond the 12-hour window with a bad diet—as I mentioned before, a diet that includes a lot of fat and sugar—they showed very poor results in terms of muscle wasting and insulin sensitivity. And when the rats ate beyond a 12-hour window with a healthier diet, they were pretty much okay, but there was no significant gain in muscle mass or improved insulin sensitivity. However, when the mice were eating a generally healthy diet *within* a 12-hour window, the result was massive improvements in muscle sparing and insulin sensitivity. When the window was reduced to just nine hours, the positive results were even greater. And what were the mice allowed to consume in the hours outside their feeding window, you might ask? Just water. Interesting right? Now let's hold that thought and discuss some widely held erroneous beliefs that need to be addressed.

The title of this chapter suggests that you should avoid intermittent fasting and this is an issue of what is popular versus what is true. As mentioned earlier time restricted eating and intermittent fasting are essentially the same. However, the main reason why I stay away from using the *term* intermittent fasting is that it is fairly trendy to start your intermittent fast on a 16:8. This means that your starting point requires you to fast for 16 hours and only eat within an 8 hour window. You will find that this book focuses on progression. Knowing what I know about the demographic I serve, I feel it would be unwise to use the term intermittent fasting knowing that your inevitable google search will encourage you to start with a 16 hour fast. You may not be there yet. Twelve hours may be enough of a challenge for you. So let's free ourselves from unrealistic demands and slowly work our way to heath. For the rest of this chapter, we will drop the phrase intermittent fasting and focus on time restricted eating.

Before we start talking more specifically about water-fasting, let me says something about muscle—both sparing and gaining muscle—because I can't tell you how many times I've had conversations with clients who told me—and this is especially true of women—that they don't want to add muscle because they don't want to get "bulky."

The truth is, you have over 600 muscles in your body, and the presence of muscle doesn't necessarily mean that you're going to be bulky. What it does do is give your body form, and shape, and it allows you to be strong and capable. When we're talking about being "toned," we're really just talking about having an adequate amount of muscle on your body and having relatively less fat.

Another question that I often get is whether or not fat turns into muscle when you exercise. And the answer is "no."

Essentially, when you exercise, you burn fat, because fat is just stored, but when you grow muscle, that muscle stays in place at all times. It's actually the fat on top of the muscle that is going to make you look bulky, or what bodybuilders call "puffy." So, your goal isn't necessarily to gain muscle as much as it is to activate a vehicle that is going to help your body burn all of that stored fat, so that you can then see the muscle that's underneath the skin.

Now that you understand more about muscle, let's get back to discussing time-restricted eating. One thing that Dr. Panda found out in his study with mice—although this hasn't been proven yet with humans—is that they could go "off course" up to two times a week and still reap the benefits of a time-restricted eating schedule. That means that if two days out of the week you go beyond the 12 hours, it is a reasonable assumption that you're still for the most part going to be okay. Which means that on weekends you can safely enjoy a later night out or attend a baseball game or take a long flight, whatever the case may be.

Well, what about my morning coffee?

Okay, so the next question I usually get at this point is, "What about black coffee in the morning?" As I mentioned before, anything other than water is going to start your clock for the day, and because coffee is xenobiotic, it's going to kick off metabolic processes in the liver and gut. The same would go for tea or herbs. Technically water with lemon counts as well, sorry! So, although it's trendy on social media to begin a fast with black coffee or to remain in your fast while drinking black coffee, doing so means that you're technically not in water fast. You may be consuming zero calories with coffee, but you're not getting the same physiological benefits (as it relates to muscle sparing) as you would if you were just consuming water. My advice, then, would be to delay that first cup of coffee *if possible,* or commit to just ending your day earlier and then consuming only water once your time-restricted eating window ends. Is drinking coffee the end of the world? No. But I would encourage you to strive for a true water fast.

Now that you understand your feeding window—what it is and what you're going to shoot for, what turns it on and what turns it off—you're probably now going to ask me, "How many calories am I supposed to consume?" And I'm going to give you an answer that is not found in any literature that's peer-reviewed but that *is* based on the 10-plus years that I've had, training clients on a practical level and seeing what's easy for them to understand, trust, implement, and also modify as their bodies start to change. In fact, you can go over to BFF Boot Camp's Instagram page to see some of the results that this method has yielded.

Finding your starting calorie target number

My main concern is that you don't consume too *few* calories. Your starting target number of calories for consumption depends on several factors, including whether you're a man or a woman, your weight, and your body fat percentage. To find the latter, you can get a body fat scale on the internet anywhere, or you can go to a testing site that measures your body fat underwater, which is the most accurate method.

We'll start with the women because most of my clients are women. If you are female and your body fat is over 33%, you'll need to multiply your weight by 9 to find your starting calorie target. If your body fat is between 24% and 33%, you'll multiply your weight by 10. And if your body fat is under 24%, you'll multiply your weight by 11.

For men, if your body fat is above 25%, you're going to multiply your weight by 9 to get your starting calorie target. If your body fat is between 12% and 24%, you'll multiply your weight by 10. And if your body fat is below 12%, you'll multiply your weight by 11.

So then, that calculation will give you the starting target number for your daily calories, and from there, you'll need to consider your activity level. The American College of Sports Medicine, at the time of my certification process, suggested that the average human engages in two to three hours a week of moderate to vigorous exercise per week. If you're getting two to three hours per week, then congratulations, you don't need to make any changes to the target daily calorie number that you just calculated for yourself. Just follow the 12-hour or, if you're able, nine-hour eating window. And I encourage you to get as close to three hours per week of exercise as possible.

Now, if you're engaging in *more than* three hours per week of moderate to vigorous exercise, you'll need to add an extra 100 calories each day for each hour you go over three hours of exercise per week. For example, if you calculated that you should consume 1500 calories based on your weight and body fat percentage, but then you work out moderately-to-vigorously six hours per week, you'll need to add 300 calories to your number. So, instead of 1500 calories, your minimum daily calories is now 1800, and that will be your goal.

With that said, for some people it may come as a shock to hear a figure like 1800 calories as a goal. What I would suggest is that you don't beat yourself up if you can't always quite get to your goal number. The most important thing is that you don't under-eat on your feeding days. So, if your goal number is supposed to be 2100 calories, but you can only get to 1900, you don't have to necessarily force feed yourself, but psychologically I just want you to remember that there is room for more calories, provided they are clean. After you go over some of the foods you should avoid, you actually my find it quite difficult to hit your number. Again, don't beat yourself up or force feed yourself. My main goal is for you to enjoy the freedom of properly fueling your body.

Now that you know how to calculate your target daily number of calories, the next question you might want to ask is, "What foods am I supposed to consume to reach this calorie number?" Again, I'll give you suggestions based on what has worked well for most people in our gym. This is information you are more than welcome to run by your primary care physician.

The standard American diet, and the diet that is most often suggested in many personal training manuals, suggests that you take in 45% to 60% of your calories from carbohydrates, around 20% to 30% of your calories from protein, and 15% to 25% of your calories from fat. However, I've found that this approach tends to lead to overconsumption of carbs in the form of sugar.

My eyes were opened on this topic when I was studying for my CrossFit Level 1 certificate. That's when I learned about the Zone Diet, which has a much simpler and what I've found to be a more effective breakdown of your recommended macronutrients. The Zone Diet allocates 40% of your calories to carbohydrates, 30% of your calories to protein, and 30% to your fat. I offer clients a margin of error of about 5%. So, if by chance you overconsume your carbohydrates, and you're at 45%, that's not the biggest deal, but the overall 40-30-30 split should be your goal.

In view of all this, when considering what you should be eating during your restricted-eating window, I generally suggest to my clients that they do their best to focus on abstaining from four things: first, avoid alcohol; second, avoid any kind of dairy; third, avoid processed carbohydrates (meaning food that has white, wheat flour, or added sugar in it); and fourth, abstain from eating or drinking *anything* (except water) outside the 12-hour window that we've been talking about.

Again, what I'm saying here is that you refrain from these things to the best of your ability. There is, of course, variation from person to person, and there are arguments that can be made for and against all kinds of food items—arguments that I'm in no position to debate because this is a training book, not a scientific journal article. But what I can tell you is that the people who have followed the easy-to-understand guidelines I just gave you have seen success, and these guidelines leave plenty of room for you to take in many different kinds of healthy foods.

Now that we've talked about what you should avoid eating and what your minimum daily calorie count should be, this is a good place to step back and remind ourselves of the purpose of this restricted-eating approach. You might be thinking, "I don't know why I can't just jump directly into a full-blown water fast," but you have to remember that going immediately to zero calories over the course of an entire day would be very difficult, especially when your body is used to consuming calories over a period of 16 to 18 hours. That's why I'm advising you first get good at restricting yourself to 12 hours, and then from there, restricting yourself to just nine or 10 hours. Once you're able to do this consistently, while still maintaining the 40-30-30 split for your macronutrients, *then* you'll then be ready to entertain the idea of a longer fast or maybe even a full-day water fast.

In the meantime, the best advice I can give you is to consume as much water as possible while you are adjusting to the 12-hour window. Your body has been conditioned to eat over and over again over the course of many years, but it doesn't have to be that way. In fact, if we look back thousands of years into history, the human body was more used to going long periods of time without food, back in our hunter and gatherer days.

So then, remember that it's probably smarter to ease into this, and just begin where you are. First, find your target-daily caloric intake number, then try to estimate the amount of time that you usually spend in your normal feeding window. Then, work that window slowly down by limiting it to one fewer hour each week. For example, if you're used to an 18-hour eating window, try to get yourself down to 17 hours the first week, and then 16 hours the next week. Keep on working yourself down until you're able to get to 12 hours, and then maybe 11, 10, and finally nine.

You have to understand that this is a process. And while some people may want to jump straight into the full-day water fast, I don't recommend it because I don't want you and your co-workers and loved ones to be miserable. Let's make this a relatively easy transition and focus first on eating healthy within a shorter window of time that you'll be maintaining between fasts. Once you have that under your belt, we can move on to full-day fasting.

For more advice on time-restricted eating from a much smarter person than me, I encourage you to search for Dr. Rhonda Patrick on YouTube and check out her YouTube page *Found My Fitness.*

Recap

Let's recap what we've covered so far and lay it out step-by-step:

1. First, consider the typical time you have your first meal or first coffee or tea of the day. Then count the number of hours between that first meal or drink until the time you normally have your last food or drink before you go to sleep. This number of hours will be the starting point for your eating window.
2. From there, you'll work on cutting back one hour each week from this eating window, until you get down to a 12-hour window, or even better, a nine-hour window.
3. After that, you're going to begin working on what you actually eat during that 12- or nine-hour window. First, you'll focus on avoiding alcohol, dairy, and processed carbohydrates, but otherwise, you're going to eat whatever you want and however much you want, but only within the window.
4. Once you've been able to do that for two weeks, staying away from those "no-go" foods, you'll determine your weight and your body fat percentage, and from those you'll calculate your target daily number of calories following the formula I gave you earlier. So, for example, if you're a man with a body fat of 24% or higher, you'll multiply your weight by nine. And if you're a woman with a body fat of 33% or higher, you'll multiply your weight by nine.

5. With your target daily number of calories in mind, you'll then aim for an overall macronutrient goal of 40% carbohydrates, 30% protein, and 30% fat. I suggest that you download the MyFitnessPal app to your phone to enter the foods you eat into your daily journal, and the app will automatically tell you what your macronutrient balance is.
6. Next, you're going to get a little more active and try to get at least two hours of moderate-to-vigorous exercise per week. If you exceed that number, remember you're going to add an extra 100 calories a day for each hour of exercise per week beyond three. And that is going to be your non-fasting diet goal from here on out.
7. Finally, while you are fasting outside your eating window, you're going to commit to drinking as much water as possible to curb your appetite. I prefer water at room temperature, but that is up to you. If you're looking for a goal number, take your weight in pounds and divide it by 2. That will be your goal number of ounces. (example, if you weigh 150lbs, your goal will be 75 ounces of water every day.) Once you've conquered your time-restricted eating goal for 30 days straight, you'll probably find that your body has already started to exhibit significant changes in the area of decreased body fat and increased energy. Congratulations!

Recap Pro Tips

- The best way to make sure you are actually hitting 40-30-30 in your diet is to make sure you are accurately entering your food quantity. To that end, I highly recommend measuring your food as you enter it into MyfitnessPal to the best of your ability. A food scale and measuring cups will ensure that you are accurate. Just remember to measure your food in its uncooked state. Your meats should be measured raw and thawed whenever possible. Your grains, like rice and oatmeal, should be measured dry.
- Be cautious with added salt. Many people add salt to their food liberally, even before they've taken their first bite. Not only does a salt addiction make portion control difficult, it also may contribute to excess water retention. Given the fact that you may be ingesting more water than you're used to, this can lead to weight gain that will falsely lead you to believe you are getting "fatter". So while salt isn't a villain here, make sure not to over consume.
- Get as much sleep a possible. Aside from sleep allowing your body time to repair, from a practical level, the more hours that you are able to sleep the fewer opportunities to you have extend your feeding window. Moreover, getting adequate sleep allows you better to control your appetite. Sleep deprived adults have higher ghrelin levels, (a hormone that increases hunger) and experiences

- less of a feeling of fullness compared to those who are able to get 7-9 hours of sleep.
- Keep your stress levels in check. I know this is no easy task, but maintaining high levels of stress on a practical and psychological level tends to encourage us to self-heal with food. On a chemical level, increased stressed releases cortisol (an insulin-antagonist hormone), which in turn, raises blood glucose levels. It can in turn increase your cravings for sweet, fatty, and salty foods. How can you control this? Practicing meditation, keeping a journal, or funding an outlet to release your stress like a boxing class.

Now it's time to entertain the idea of full day fasting. Which we will discuss in chapter 2.

Chapter Two

How we Burn Fat and Therapeutic Fasting

In Chapter One I gave you some actionable tasks to repeat during your eating windows, complete with target daily calories, time restrictions, and foods that you'll want to definitely stay away from. However, if you are like a lot of my clients, you may have either skipped Chapter One or looked at the information and disregarded it, saying to yourself that you've tried something like that already and you just want to get straight to the fasting.

Given that possibility, I want to start this Therapeutic Fasting chapter by explaining what goes on inside your body if you choose to deviate from the water fast or if you do what a lot of people do and try to simply eat the fewest number of calories possible or, as it's sometimes called, "eating in moderation"—instead of aiming for your target caloric intake number while staying within your eating window as I explained in Chapter One.

A lot of these harmful dieting habits have been reinforced by shows like *The Biggest Loser*, which has been the bane of my existence since I started training. Of course, it's a great representation of how *not* to diet if you want to see long-term success. You probably already know that the show revolves around morbidly obese people who spend time on a ranch with trainers, where they significantly decrease the number of calories they consume while doing excessively difficult workouts. Weekly, they hop on a scale to see how much weight they've lost. And it's great for television when you see the average contestant lose 10, 7, or 15 pounds in a "week."

Now, we understand, of course, that this show is made for TV, and anything made for TV is geared toward getting ratings, so that during the commercials you can buy the products shown in the ads. Nothing that happens on *The Biggest Loser* is all that realistic anyway; so, for example, what they may call "a week" might actually be longer, like 10 to 14 days—maybe it's more time; maybe it's less, we'll never know. The show also never clearly points out that given the contestants' extreme state of obesity, they're experiencing a much higher caloric deficit, which allows them to lose weight faster than most people can. It's also worth pointing out that these people are on a ranch and have the luxury of ignoring everything related to work or family responsibilities, which won't be the case for most people trying to lose weight. The point is that with this show you're getting a false idea of what a realistic weight loss goal should be over the course of a week.

But you might notice a couple of other things about this show. First, isn't it odd that when the contestants get relatively close to regular obesity, where most people are right now, the show sends the clients home for about four months to finish losing the last 30 or 40 pounds on their own? Have you ever wondered why they do that? Another thing that you might notice is that they never have a reunion show for *The Biggest Loser*. Have you ever wondered why not?

Well, the reason they don't show the client losing those last 30 or 40 pounds is that it would be extremely boring to show this on TV, because the rate of fat loss after those initial months on the show, once the contestants go home, will be much, much slower. At that point they're probably losing maybe two to four pounds a week, and that's a lot closer to what you're probably going to experience too if everyone in your circle is doing everything to accommodate your fitness goals and you have $100,000 on the line. Spoiler alert, they won't, and you don't.

But the saddest part about *The Biggest Loser* is the fact that they never have reunion shows. And that's mainly because most of the participants are required to sign a nondisclosure agreement stating that for a period of time after the show is over, they can't talk about their sustained fat loss. And this is because in most cases, they *don't* sustain the fat loss. Let me explain why.

If you follow *The Biggest Loser's* "eat less, move more" model and then just continually cut your calories to the point of 1200 or even below 1000 calories, you'll certainly lose weight over time. But you might as well think of this weight loss as fool's gold, because at the same time you're losing weight, you're also hurting your metabolism by slowing it down. What I mean is, as you keep losing weight, your basal metabolic rate—which is the number of calories your body burns without you moving at all—also decreases over time. So, the number of calories necessary to continue weight loss keeps on decreasing over time, to the point where you will be literally starving yourself to lose weight and operating with an inefficient body.

For instance, a client who might have come on *The Biggest Loser* show burning 1800 calories a day may work themselves down to the point where they're burning only 1200 calories a day because they've been continually underfeeding their body. But that is going to force them to eat fewer and fewer calories, and *that* is not a healthy lifestyle.

Instead, your goal should be to maintain your basal metabolic rate over the course of your weight-loss journey. In fact, if possible, you'll want to *increase* your metabolic rate so you can eat more while still losing weight. This is a common "problem" that my clients happily experience after they've turned their bodies into fat-burning machines and have to eat more just to maintain their weight.

So now let's just jump into why your body stores fat and how you can flip that switch off. Before I go into explaining this, I first have to give a lot of credit to Dr. Jason Fung, who created a video on YouTube entitled *Therapeutic Fasting*, in which he tries to solve the "two-compartment problem."

Dr. Fung explains that whenever you eat foods, you increase insulin. And what is insulin? Insulin is a hormone that signals the body to store sugar in the liver, produce fat in the liver, and store that fat.

When you consume carbohydrates, they're essentially metabolized as glucose, and glucose will be your readily available form of energy. All the excess glucose you consume is stored as glycogen, which is like a backup form of energy for your body to access. When you have too much glycogen in your body, your liver produces lipids, which basically store fat in the body.

So then, when you don't eat, essentially your insulin levels fall, and that's a trigger to start pulling some of the stored energy out in the form of glycogen. Once you've depleted both your glucose and your glycogen, as long as your insulin levels are low, then your body can opt for stored fat as its secondary source of energy.

Dr. Fung makes a very easy-to-understand comparison: Your glycogen is like the refrigerator that's immediately available to you in your kitchen. And your stored fat is like your freezer, which is over in your basement or in the garage. So, the glycogen, which is in your body's "refrigerator," is much easier to access as energy. The freezer, however, which is in the garage or basement, requires a lot more energy to pull out of. Your body's "freezer" is going to be storing the fat.

Now, your "refrigerator" has a limited capacity, meaning that your body can only store so much glycogen. When you reach a surplus of glycogen, your body is automatically going to bypass the "refrigerator" and put everything in the "freezer," which is the fat storage.

So then, overconsumption of carbohydrates without burning them off and without an adequate amount of fasting time is going to lead to constant storage of fat. When you look at the body as a two-compartment storage system, with both an easy to access "refrigerator" and a harder to access "freezer," things start to make a lot of sense. If instead it was a one-compartment system, and all of the stored sugar and stored fat went to the same place, it would make sense that all you have to do is decrease calories and you would automatically decrease fat.

But that's not the case: Your body is selective as to which sources of energy it chooses to use for fuel. And your main goal needs to be to try to pull the fat energy out as much as possible.

Now, the main thing that controls whether or not we are pulling fat from the freezer or just glycogen from the refrigerator is the level of insulin, which is essentially going to be the traffic control system of your body, dictating the energy source that your body burns for fuel. One of the main jobs of insulin is to limit lipolysis, which basically means that insulin prevents you from taking the fat out of the freezer. So, when your insulin level is high, like when you have a large meal, or maybe constant meals throughout the day, you're preventing your body from reaching into the freezer and using fat as a form of energy.

Here's where "eating everything in moderation" goes wrong. If you continue to eat multiple times a day, every day with your carb-heavy(+50% of your calories with very little fiber) diet, and not enough physical activity, you're not in any way lowering the effects of insulin. Insulin is still going to do its job, which is to store fat. The only thing that you're doing by taking fewer and fewer calories is signaling to your body that it needs to *burn* fewer and fewer calories. So, when you eat less and your insulin stays high, you just burn fewer calories.

The point of fasting is to turn insulin off so lipolysis is not blocked and your body will now rely on the energy(in the form of fat) from the freezer. Your body must first burn up the available glucose and glycogen before it can access your stare fat as energy. The body will now target specifically the fat in the freezer as its form of energy.

When that happens, you can now consider your stored fat— since it's being used as fuel during your fast—as your "calories in," because that's what your body is burning. And because the fat is available in abundance, you cannot starve yourself. Mentally you might feel like you need to eat, in the shorter-term fasts, you are in virtually no danger. The body is going to take exactly what it needs, from your storage, and it will have no need to decrease calories out and slow down your metabolism.

If we go back to the time-restricted eating that we implemented in Chapter One, you are now spending a minimum of 12 hours with a decreased insulin level. And that allows the body more time to pull from the freezer, aka the fat. As we move our way into the full-day water fast, your insulin levels are just turned off for a longer period of time, which allows the body more time to pull even more fat out of the body.

I hope now you can see the difference between eating a low number of calories throughout your entire day, which keeps insulin in play, and not consuming any calories for periods of time throughout the day, which takes insulin out of the equation entirely and allows your body to burn fat.

But what about my muscle?

The biggest concern that I hear in response to the notion of water fasting is the fear of losing muscle. Here is why you don't need to worry about that.

Kevin Hall published a study in the NIH (National Institutes of Health), where he documented the oxidation rate (or the burn rate) of carbs, proteins, and fats. He found that in muscle there was some oxidation of protein—aka amino acids—within the first 24 hours; however, that number decreased substantially at around the 30-hour mark. The same is true for carbohydrates, which at around the 30- to 36-hour mark is near zero because by then you'll have burned out all of your carbohydrates(glucose and glycogen). The interesting thing, however, is that your rate of fat burning will be triple or even quadruple the rate of carbohydrate or protein burning by the 24- to 36-hour mark. So, once you're in a fasted state for that long, your body is operating, primarily, by burning its existing, stored fat.

The reason this happens is because the body really only has two forms of energy: carbohydrates and fat. Protein is not a source of energy—it's simply a building block for tissues. So, the body will not opt to burn protein when you aren't eating in your fasted state; it will instead go for your stored body fat, which is an abundant source of preferred energy for the body once carbohydrates have been depleted. Now problems can arise if you have no glucose, glycogen, or fat. But we will soon cover who should NOT fast.

So now, I want you to visualize your two-compartment system. You already know that there is fat in your body. Now, if you don't consume calories, essentially your refrigerator is empty, so there is no form of glucose to be used as energy. You will, after about a day, have oxidized all your glycogen, which was easy to access, and your body will need its energy. At that point, it's going to reach for that stored form of energy that you carry around with you every day—your stored fat. We're essentially built to withstand periods of famine. It is only in the last few hundred years that we have had food so readily available at all times. Centuries ago, we had to hunt and gather. Our bodies needed a mechanism to withstand extended periods of time with no food. We're simply activating this mechanism.

This mechanism will initiate ketosis. Ketosis is a process where your body makes ketones. Ketones, a fatty acid, are released from the liver into the bloodstream and we use them as fuel to drive the body's metabolism and support muscle function. In a shorter fast of up to 18 hours, you will only barely start to activate ketosis. But as your water fasts span across multiple days you will release more ketones at a high rate.

But before you put this book down and swear food off for the rest of your life, let's explore who probably should not be fasting. Full-day fasting, for the purpose of this book, is not advised for people with a low BMI(below 18.5), an existing eating disorder, or pregnant people without the intervention of their primary health provider.

Side note: Your BMI (body mass index) is a measure that uses your height and weight to determine if your weight is healthy. The BMI calculation divides your weight in kilograms by your height in meters squared. But instead of doing the math yourself, you can simply Google "my BMI" and make sure your calculated number isn't below 18.5.

Also, based on what I've seen, I would advise that you don't attempt a fast while on your period, as it can be a bit too much on the mind. So, if you fall into any of these categories for which fasting is contraindicated, I would advise you to first consult your primary care physician. And it may be a better idea in such cases simply to focus only on time-restricted eating because that's still a form of water fasting—it's just a little less extreme.

Now that you understand how water fasting works, how fat burning works, how muscle burning works, and how your basal metabolic rate will be positively affected by water fasting—how often should you do it?

For most people, adjusting to time-restricted eating will be a challenge compared to their previous form of dieting. For many, the transition from time-restricted eating to full-day fasting was equally challenging, if not more so.

So, instead of jumping into the deep end of the pool, I'd suggest taking baby steps. The best thing that you can do is pick one day out of the week to practice something that is commonly referred to as OMAD, which is an acronym for "One Meal a Day." With this approach, you'll be on an advanced regular time-restricted eating schedule. You're going to pick one day to operate on an 18+hour fast.

The question then is what meals should you skip for this longer fast? Breakfast and lunch? Lunch and dinner? I'll leave that up to you because I've heard from various people that different times of the day work better for them. I personally prefer to skip breakfast and dinner. So, my one meal is in the early afternoon. No matter which meals you skip, you're essentially going to give yourself a one-hour window in which you'll consume your one meal for that day, and the remainder of the day will be water fasting. Keep in mind, this is not the time to order Chinese food, or to severely spike your insulin with a large piece of cake. If you feel the need to have unusually unhealthy food for your one meal, you aren't ready for OMAD.

Another approach to consider is alternate-day fasting. With this method, you have one day in which you completely water fast, then the next day you have your regular meals and caloric intake, and then you keep on alternating days in this way. For those who are obese (BMI +30), this approach can prove to be very beneficial, and it can also be maintained for extended periods of time, up to 30 days or more of alternate day fasting.

You can also choose to use the OMAD method for your fasting days. If you decide to use that approach, the only caveat is that you should keep the one meal under 500 calories, because that way your body will still think you're fasting and will continue to function as if you are.

I would suggest coming up with an OMAD meal that you'll enjoy, not high in sugar, and that ideally falls close to the "40% carbohydrates, 30% protein, 30% fat" ratio. And if you want to take things a step further, you can actually have a "higher fat (50%), lower carb (30%), moderate protein (20%)" meal on your fasting day, so that your body will have much less glucose and glycogen to burn. An omelet with avocado and a cup of berries would be a great example of a higher fat meal that still gives you carbs and protein.

Again, you may be incline to commit to alternate day fasting immediately, but we always recommend baby steps. Try OMAD once a week for three weeks. Afterwards, pick two OMAD days for two weeks. Once that becomes easy, you can try alternate-day fasting for another three weeks. Once you feel comfortable with this, perhaps one of the three OMAD days can become a straight water fast, with no meal at all on that day.

Essentially, you'll be creating a step program for yourself. And once you're able to successfully get through a full day of water fasting without going crazy or assaulting your co-workers, you'll know that you're prepared for the next level. In the next chapter, we'll go over what it means to stack multiple days of water-only fasts up to 48 hours, and we'll see what that does for your body, chemically.

Now, before and during your water fast, there is one piece of advice that you absolutely have to follow: *Do not consume distilled water on water fasts*. Distilled water is going to be horrible for you. While you're fasting, you will be in a situation where you are not eating, and distilled water can essentially further strip your body of its minerals. So, you want to make sure to stick with spring water while you're fasting, to stay safe.

Now that we're practicing entire water-fasting days or days in which our caloric intake has been lowered enough to simulate fasting, it's especially important to remember that you're consuming enough water, taking half of your weight in pounds, then replacing the "pounds" with "ounces," and that becomes your daily goal for how many ounces of water to drink.

So, if you weigh 200 pounds, your goal would be to consume at least 100 ounces of water a day, whether you're on a time-restricted eating schedule, an OMAD, or a complete water fast. I tend to consume a little bit more water to keep my mind busy while I'm doing a water-only fast. But half your weight in ounces should be your absolute minimum to start.

And once again, I want to reiterate that anybody who has a low BMI should abstain from water fasting if they don't have the okay from their primary care physician. Likewise, pregnant women should abstain from water-only fasting, and people who suffer from anorexia or bulimia should avoid water-only fasting. Again, anybody who qualifies for water-only fasting should be consuming at least half their weight in ounces of water and should tread the idea of full-day fasting very slowly and gradually.

Recap

Let's recap the step program covered in this chapter for introducing the OMAD and the 24-hour water fast.

1. First, before you begin actually cutting out entire meals, you'll want to make sure that time-restricted eating has become easy for you and that you're no longer as reliant on consuming copious amounts of carbohydrates in excess of 45% of your calories on any given day. This includes the fact that if you do go beyond your nine- to 12-hour feeding window, this happens no more than two times a week.
2. Once you've mastered time-restricted eating, you're now going to pick one day out of the week that is best for you for the OMAD technique. Some people prefer to do this on their busiest day of the week; others thrive best when they do their OMAD on days when they don't have a lot going on. You'll know what feels

right for you. For that day, you're going to put together a meal with absolutely no more than 45% carbohydrates and no more than 500 calories. And you are going to consume that meal within one hour, so that you'll essentially be fasting for 18+ hours straight twice in a relatively short amount of time. Your insulin will drop to near zero towards the end of your OMAD, which means you'll have enjoyed the benefits of a full-day simulated fast.

3. Once this has become relatively easy to do, you can then take one of two routes: Option One would be to begin doing OMAD for two days out of the week instead of just one, and then eventually expand it to three days out of the week and alternate between the 12- or nine-hour restricted-eating days and the OMAD simulated-fast days. You could then continue this schedule for as long as you like and as long as your health remains at an optimal level, physically, emotionally, and psychologically.

4. Option Two would be to take the one OMAD per week you've been doing and go ahead and replace it with a full 24-hour day of water fasting, where no food is consumed, just water. Once you're comfortable with that schedule, you could then introduce a second OMAD day into your weekly schedule, which would later likewise be replaced by another full 24-hour day of fasting, and so forth. Again, you could then continue this schedule for as long as your body remains in good health, physically, emotionally, and psychologically.

5. Bear in mind, as mentioned before with the time-restricted eating, that if you're doing the OMAD, coffee does count. So, in an ideal situation, you'd consume your coffee within that same hour that you're going to have your meal.
6. If your main goal is overall weight loss, then either of the two approaches just explained should be enough to see you through to a healthy BMI and healthy body fat percentage. Just make sure to do your best to get two hours of moderate to vigorous physical activity every week. Vigorous workouts should be avoided on your water fasting only days. As an alternative to vigorous exercise, you can go for a walk or do yoga.

Remember, if your main goal is weight loss, and you seeing success with the OMAD coupled with a 9-hour time restricted eating schedule. Just keep doing it. The goal of fat loss and weight loss is to find something that works. If you find something that works that can be sustained over an extended period of time, success is inevitable.

For those of you who want explore increased benefits of water fasting, the idea of stacking fasting days will be your next adventure. This also will apply to people who have a chronic disease and want to put their body in a position to better cope with their illness. In the next chapter we'll talk about the benefits of stacking water fasts over multiple days for up to 48 hours.

Chapter Three

The 48-Hour Fast

Congratulations on successfully implementing the practice of time restricted eating from Chapter 1. Through this effort, you have decreased the amount of stored glycogen in the body, which has made it easier for your body to access the stored body fat; you also decreased your blood glucose; and you started to increase your blood ketone levels.

Once you've started implementing time-restricted eating coupled with an OMAD, which we discussed in chapter 2, you've further increased your body's ability to burn fat. You've also created a measurable uptick in your ketone bodies. And the ketones do more than just burn fat; they're hormones that signal a decrease in inflammation, an increase in DNA repair, and an increase in something called human growth hormone or HGH, as well as an increase in BDNF, which is a brain-derived neurotrophic factor.

HGH and BDNF together are extremely important for the brain because they're important for cell repair and strengthening neural connections. This means you'll be able to make better and stronger neural networks every time you learn something. An increase in HGH and BDNF will also aid in cartilage growth and repair for your sore joints, and it can actually improve immune cell function. So, just by fasting for 18 hours, you're creating a lot of beneficial physiological changes within the body.

Now, one thing to consider is that the benefits you experience from an 18-hour fast—the decreased inflammation, increased DNA repair, and the increased HGH and BDNF—are also improved when you exercise. So, exercising is only going to accelerate this. This is not to say that you should just exercise or you should just fast. Essentially, when you're able incorporate both habits into your lifestyle, you're getting the best of both worlds, and you're having your body operate at its peak capability.

Once you're able to go beyond the 18-hour mark into a full-day, 24-hour water fast, you'll start to experience something very exciting called *autophagy*. What is autophagy, you ask? Well, the term translates directly as "cell death." Autophagy, as defined by the National Cancer Institute, is a process by which a cell breaks down and destroys old, damaged, or abnormal proteins and other substances in its cytoplasm (the fluid inside the cell). The breakdown products are then recycled for important cell functions, especially during periods of stress or starvation. Autophagy also helps destroy bacteria and viruses that cause infection, and it may prevent normal cells from becoming cancer cells. Autophagy may also affect the body's immune response against viruses, bacteria, and cancer cells.

In layman's terms, when your body is well-fed, it has an abundance of resources from which it can pull for energy. However, when you stop feeding the body, the body has to become more selective with its resources. Not all of the cells in the body are equally essential. So, if you are low on energy and your body needs to create more energy, the body will, in essence, start to thrive off of itself. The cells that you have in your body that are not as beneficial to the body, perhaps some autoimmune cells, will be the first ones to be martyred as your body maintains its health. So then, at the 24-hour mark, you're now starting to affect your body on a cellular level. And that's where things get really exciting.

Now, what happens when you've been water fasting for 48 hours? Your body will continue the process of autophagy, where you're essentially eliminating cells that are less healthy, less efficient, and less essential for you to operate at an optimal level. You're also increasing your ketone bodies, which means that you're burning more fat for energy over the course of the 48 hours. You're also increasing your BDNF, where you'll now be able to make stronger neural connections, and you're increasing your human growth hormone at a rate of 500%—which means you're making five times as much growth hormone as you did before and therefore are, essentially, five times more effective with fatty acid utilization, protein synthesis, amino acid transport, immune cell function, cartilage growth, collagen synthesis, and the retention of electrolytes such as nitrogen, sodium, potassium, phosphorus. All of this is improved fivefold when you water fast for 48 hours as opposed to 24 hours. And at this point, you're also continuing to decrease inflammation.

But wait, there's more. Do you remember when we previously discussed basal metabolic rate? That's the rate at which your body burns calories at rest. At around the 48-hour mark, you'll actually start to see an increase in your basal metabolic rate by up to 10%. You know how you keep saying, your metabolism is slowing down because you're getting older? Well, now you have a way to combat that.

So, the question now is, how do you get there? Going two straight days without consuming anything but water is going to be a challenge, but there are some things you can do to make achieving your 48-hour fast easier.

For instance, if you have a very heavy carbohydrate and sugar-based diet going into your fast, you're going to find it uncomfortable to transition from using glycogen and glucose as your main source of energy to burning fat as your main source of energy. In that case, you may experience the same kinds of symptoms you would if you were to work out on an empty stomach, symptoms such as lightheadedness, dizziness, or nausea. However, once you are in ketosis, you'll find that your hunger pains decrease significantly.

So, the transition to fat burning through ketones can be made easier if you do it first with food and get your body to a point where it is already burning fat for fuel before you remove entirely the fat intake from the body. How can you do this? By tapering yourself off of your time-restricted eating diet and consuming a diet for a day or two that is comprised mostly of fat. This is essentially the ketogenic diet. And while I personally am not a proponent of the ketogenic diet long-term for fat loss, I have found that it makes it easier to transition into the fasting mode when your body is already burning fat for fuel, which is the end goal of the water fast anyway.

This ketogenic transition can be accomplished by switching your macronutrient breakdown from 40% carbs, 30% protein, and 30% fat to more of a ketogenic breakdown of 70% fat, no more than 20% protein, and no more than 10% carbohydrates. It's actually best if you have about 75% fat, and then about 15% to 20% protein, and 5% to 10% carbohydrates.

Most of your diet during this fatty phase will consist, then, of fat-based items such as eggs, nuts, seeds, and avocados. And instead of the leaner proteins, like chicken breasts, you'll transition over to fattier forms of protein such as salmon or steak. You can cook your eggs with ghee in order to increase the amount of fat that you're taking in, and also replace your oatmeal with a chia pudding, where you put half a cup of chia seeds into unsweetened coconut milk and let them soak overnight so that the mixture has thickened up by the next day(feel free to add your favorite berry and a tbsp of monkfruit sweetener for taste). The body will start to rely more on fat as its source of fuel.

In this way, when you start your water fast, your body will already be used to burning fat as its main source of energy, making the shock of going from sugar to fat for energy not so drastic.

Decreasing or eliminating your intake of the following foods while preparing to fast may make the attainment of a ketogenic state and the transition into a 48 hour fast a little bit easier: whole grains, rice, oatmeal, fruit, starchy vegetables, and beans. The one thing you want to remember to do is make this transition gradually, so that just in case you have any negative effects, you can very easily transition back to your regular form of eating. At that point it may be better to enlist the advice of you registered dietician or primary care provider. Instead of going straight from 40% carbohydrates to 5% carbohydrates, then, you can have a couple of days in between where you go from 40% carbohydrates, 30% protein, and 30% fat to, say, 20% carbohydrates, 30% protein, and 50% fat, and then finally 10% carbohydrates, 20% protein, and 70% fat. And as long as you don't see any adverse effects, you can continue on with your ketogenic lead into your water fast.

The next thing you'll want to do is make sure to hyperhydrate: Drink a lot of water before you start your longer fasts, mainly because you don't want to dehydrate yourself. Going into a fast dehydrated is only going to make you hungrier, so you want to make sure that you don't set yourself up for failure as you start your water fast.

In addition to that, you want to make sure that you get a lot of minerals into the body because when you operate on only water, especially if you're aiming for a +48-hour fast, you may experience a loss of minerals. One product that I like is an electrolyte drink or electrolyte tablets. There's a company I found on Amazon called Nuun that sells these. (I'm not being sponsored by them, by the way.) It's simply an effervescent electrolyte supplement that you can put into your water as you're hydrating right before you start your fast, in order to make sure that you are filled with minerals. It's also a good idea while you're doing your keto diet and preparing for your fast that you get multivitamins in your system.

The point is that you want to: number one, be hydrated as you go into your fast, and number two, make sure you have minerals in your system, including sodium, potassium, and calcium.

Now, let's talk about exercise. Engaging in a high-intensity workout while you're low in blood sugar and still not yet in ketogenesis may not yield the best results for you. Lower-intensity alternatives to consider include walking, Pilates, tai chi, or yoga. During your one or two days of a water fast, these will be a welcome break from your normal high intensity exercise and will promote recovery, repair, and relaxation. Remember, the body is a tool that thrives not only on work but also on rest. So, you don't need to do 100 burpees in order to see success while you're fasting.

If you're looking for one more benefit of a water fast that lasts 24 - 48 hours, consider gut healing. Our gut microbiome essentially resets about every three days. And if we're constantly inundating it with food, we're not necessarily giving our gut a chance to rest and recover. Giving your gut one or two days off allows the gut lining to reset.

I've decided to save the best benefit for last as it relates to fasting. And it's the benefit that I'm sure most people who purchase this book will enjoy most. It's this: Once you're fasting beyond 24 hours, you're going to find that the body selectively chooses to burn fat around the midsection. How cool is that?

In fact, one thing you might find during your 24-48-hour fast is that you start to get a little cold in your extremities—in your feet, your arms, and your hands. Part of what's happening is a migration of blood from the extremities to the organs where the visceral fat is located to protect your organs. So, as this migration of blood over to your midsection occurs, it's going to create a thermogenic effect, and this heat burns fat around the midsection more so than around your arms and legs.

Moreover, keep in mind that we have billions of bacteria in our biome, not all of which are friendly bacteria. So, giving the gut an opportunity to rest and recover is going to be extremely beneficial while you're doing your two-day fast. This is especially true because you will not be consuming as much sugar, a substance that many of our not so friendly bacteria thrives on.

Breaking your fast

Now, the main issue that a lot of people are going to have, is how to break their 48-hour fast effectively. You need to exercise a little bit more caution when breaking a 48 hour fast as opposed to an 18 or 24 hour fast. When you begin to eat again, it's kind of like waking your body up from a deep sleep. Imagine if you were sleeping and somebody was going to wake you up, you wouldn't want them to throw an entire bucket of cold water on you; you'd want them to perhaps play a soft sound, and then a slightly louder sound, and then maybe shake you a little bit.

Similarly, if you allow yourself to get completely ravenous during your fast and then break it with something very rich, especially something high in sugar, your gastrointestinal response may be less than ideal. So, the first thing you're going to want to do is make sure that you keep your hunger under control during a fast. And when it's time to break it, you won't have allowed yourself to become ravenous. You want to be minimally hungry so that you can give yourself about 12 to 24 hours of fast breaking.

This is how you're going to do it: After two days of consuming no food, your body will be operating in ketosis. You'll have probably burned through all your glucose and stored glycogen, so your body will be running on fat. With that in mind, you're going to start breaking your fast by giving yourself foods that have the same energy signature as what your body has been using. So, you'll want to have some MCT oil on hand and give yourself one or two tablespoons at a time, perhaps spread about three hours apart, and that's going to be a good way to give you a quick energy boost and begin reintroducing foods into your system.

The MCT oil will also help you to start to feel satisfied, like you've actually eaten food. Even though you'll still be a little hungry, you won't have the strong hunger pangs. Another benefit of consuming MCT oil is that it relaxes you out without raising your insulin level, so you'll remain in ketosis and still be experiencing the benefits of the fast. And autophagy, which is the body getting rid of cells that you don't need, will continue as well, as long as you don't start consuming protein. By initially sticking with foods that are primarily fat as you begin breaking your fast, you can stay within autophagy.

Now then, 3 to 6 hours after you've consumed your first MCT oil, you'll want to focus on repopulating the gut with very good bacteria so it can start to function again at an optimal level. While you were fasting, a fair amount of the bacteria in your system died off, some good and some bad, so now is your opportunity to put good bacteria back into your system. Your best food options to repopulate your gut with good bacteria are fermented foods.

You *could* go the route of taking probiotics, but foods that have been through the actual fermentation process will be better. One of your best options is sauerkraut, which is a fermented food. You can also go with my personal favorite, kimchi: It's a fermented blend of cabbage and other vegetables and can be quite spicy as well, if you like spice.

You could also go the route of yogurt, but if you do, it shouldn't have any fruit in it, and it shouldn't even be vanilla flavored. The yogurt that you want to consume after your fast will actually be very sour. When yogurt is sweet, that's usually a clear sign that it won't have the same positive effects on your good bacteria, because you're consuming not only food that will feed the good bacteria but also the fruit and/or syrup—which is absolutely not good for you and feeds the bad bacteria as well. So, to be on the safe side, yogurt will probably not be the best option during the first day or two of breaking your fast, when you want to make sure that you're feeding your body as ideally as possible and repopulating the gut.

After you've started off breaking your fast with fermented foods, then you can start to reintroduce other solid foods into your diet in the form of steamed veggies or perhaps a vegetable soup with a low amount of salt. These will give your body the fuel and the fiber that you need to feed the good bacteria. So, sauerkraut, kimchi, and—to a lesser degree—yogurt is going to repopulate the gut with good bacteria, and the steamed vegetables and vegetable soup will feed the good bacteria that you have repopulated.

The next thing to add into your fast-breaking routine is bone broth, which is vital for realigning the gut and further feeding your biome. There are a lot of benefits when it comes to consuming bone broth. Gelatin is the most abundant protein in bone broth. Once it enters your digestive tract, gelatin binds with water to support healthy digestion. Also, collagen, which is a byproduct of chicken bone broth has been found to improve pain, stiffness, and joint function in osteoarthritis patients. For these reasons, it may be a great idea to include bone broth as a regular part of your diet after your fast. However, the one thing that you have to remember is that bone broth will absolutely break the fast, and whatever affects you were getting from autophagy, in terms of getting rid of the auto-immune cells or less effective cells, will halt. So, while bone broth is going to be a great option to bring you back closer to regular eating, consuming it will be the point where the fast is officially broken. You'll continue to keep your insulin low, but the autophagy will cease.

The next part of your fast braking process will be to provide your body with easy to digest fibers which will act as food for your healthy bacteria. Steamed vegetables or a low sodium vegetable soup will provide your body with pre-biotics.

The last part of the fast-breaking process is to introduce foods that will support growth, and these are going to be your lean proteins, preferably pasture-raised eggs, grass-fed meat, and lean chicken. If you can get these items directly from a farm, that would be ideal, because especially as you're breaking the fast, you want to get the highest quality of these foods into your system. You can also add avocados—so, an omelet with avocados would be a fantastic option at this point. Chicken soup would be another great option depending on the time of day. And be sure, to the best of your ability, to get the highest quality beef available to you.

Finally, you can start to transition back into your zone diet by taking your macros from 75% carbs 20% protein and 5% fat back to 40% carbs 30% protein, and 30% fat. From there you can resume your time restricted eating schedule until you are ready to fast again

Recap

To wrap up this chapter, let's go over once more the benefits of water fasting for 48 hours:

1. You're going to increase your human growth hormone production by 500%, and you'll continue to increase BDNF as well.
2. You will also produce ketones, where your body runs on stored fat as fuel.
3. You will increase autophagy as well, which gets rid of cells that are not serving your body as well as others and allows your body to create new, healthier cells.
4. The extended fast will keep your insulin levels low and give your body an opportunity to decrease inflammation.
5. At this point, your stored glucose and glycogen will be at zero or pretty close to it.

In short, there are a myriad of benefits at the 48-hour mark.

In terms of breaking your fast, to make things simple, you may want to proceed in two to three intervals:

1. To begin breaking your fast, consume the MCT oil.
2. Then a few hours later, repopulate your gut with fermented foods that have good bacteria, which will be your sauerkraut, kimchi, or a very sour, unsweetened, unflavored yogurt.
3. After a few more hours, consume steamed vegetables or a vegetable soup.
4. Then a few hours after that, you can start consuming solid foods that are not vegetables. For the most part, these will still need to be very low in sugar, so good options might be chicken vegetable soup or a soup with beef in it, and if you're breaking fast in the

morning or late morning, you might choose an omelet cooked in ghee butter or with coconut oil, topped with your favorite protein and avocado.
5. After that, you can resume your previous time-restricted eating schedule.

That covers your first 48-hour fast. In the next chapter, we'll go over what happens if you're able to maintain a third day for a 72-hour fast.

Chapter Four

The 72-Hour Fast:
Unlocking Your Body's Ability to Heal Itself

Once you've gone into the third day of water fasting and hit the 72-hour mark, your body will still be experiencing the benefits that it had experienced from the 24-hour fast, including the decrease in glucose and glycogen and the onset of ketones, and it will continue experiencing the benefits of the 48-hour fast as well, which includes the increase of HGH and BDNF, the onset of autophagy, and the increase of ketone bodies in the system that allows your body to use its stored fat as energy. You'll also have begun to experience cartilage repair and increased muscle sparing.

However, at the 72-hour mark things start to get really interesting, because your body will begin to create stem cells, which are essentially the body's raw materials: cells from which all other cells with specialized functions are generated. These stem cells can become anything that your body needs, as all the tissues that make up organs start off as stem cells.

So, for instance, if you have scar tissue in the skin, stem cells will grow; the body can then use these stem cells to create new skin cells. Or if a certain organ needs healing, then the body can allocate the stem cells to creating the tissues that will help that specific organ heal. As you can see, stem cells are a very big deal when it comes to healing your body.

As I mentioned earlier, for the purposes of your health and safety, this book will not recommend that you extend your water fast beyond 72 hours. That's mainly because you would experience no new adaptations as you went into your fourth and fifth day of fasting. What you'd experience is only a slight increase of all markers, but there would be a point of diminishing returns. So, for example, your human growth hormone would not keep going up to 700%, 800%, or 900%—it would essentially stay at the 500% level it had already reached, and you'd just be producing that for a longer a period of time.

If your main goal, then, is to increase autophagy and growth hormones, and to activate the creation of more stem cells, you're going to get this done right at the 72-hour mark. If you do want to extend your fast slightly beyond 72 hours, then you could simply plan ahead by starting your fast close to bedtime, so that when you hit the 72-hour mark, it won't be hard to go to sleep, and then you'll have earned yourself an extra six to eight hours of fast while sleeping, before you break your fast the next morning (and anyway, fasting while sleeping is a natural kind of fast). Otherwise, it would behoove you to stop at 72 hours, and then repeat the fast later at an interval that is right for you.

There is another benefit to the 72-hour fast that I haven't yet mentioned: A fast of this length will help you to forget your body's old set points. So, the first thing you may experience when you break the fast is a reset of your palate, where foods that used to be mild to you, after fasting will taste very sweet or very salty. You'll also help your body to forget its old set points in terms of weight. Many of my clients have expressed to me that they hit a certain number on the scale and they can't lose any more weight. Almost as if their body is fighting them. I tend to agree that there may be some truth to that. Your body doesn't know if you're losing weight for a wedding or for sickness. So, the body in its infinite wisdom has set points that is strives to maintain in order to keep you alive. You may drop 15lbs, going from 150lbs to 135lbs, but the body's set point may cause you to gain a lot of that back only because it's used to being 150lbs and that is where it knows it's safe. So, when you reset your set points, you'll feel less of an inclination to gorge yourself and eat until you end up at your old weight. In short, your body won't fight you as you maintain good habits, and you won't find yourself plateauing and stuck the same way that you used to get stuck on the scale.

So, the next question is, "How often should I be doing a 72-hour fast?" The truth is that just about anyone can benefit from an occasional 72-hour fast, and for a healthy person without any ongoing chronic illness, whereas you may do a 24-hour fast once a month or more, you'll probably want to reserve a 72-hour fast for just once a season. If instead you are someone with an ongoing chronic illness that you're trying to resolve and your main goal is healing, then it may be in your best interest to do your 72-hour fast more often than that—as often as you feel you can handle, assuming that you are not at risk due to pregnancy, or too low of a body weight, or an eating disorder. So, the answer is that it's really up to you, and how your body feels over time will dictate whether or not this intervention is your best option.

The one thing to remember, however, is that even at the lowest level of time-restricted eating, you will receive many of the same benefits of a 12- and 18-hour fasts just by exercising, including the increase in human growth hormone, the increase in BDNF, and the decrease in inflammation. So, while you're between fasts, it's going to be very important to exercise two to three times a week to make sure that you're doing everything you need to do to keep your body as healthy as possible.

Lastly, in regard to the process of breaking a 72-hour fast, it won't really vary from the two-day process described in the preceding chapter on "The 48-hour Fast." You'll essentially follow the same guidelines for breaking your fast, where every three to six hours you'll introduce a new kind of element to the body to properly refeed the gut biome.

So then, those are the basic facts you need to know about the 72-hour fast. Much of the credit for this information can be awarded to Dr. Sten Ekberg, who has an amazing YouTube channel filled with even more information that will help you navigate your two and three-day fasts. I highly recommend that you follow Dr. Ekberg for more information on how to be successful.

Chapter Five

The Only Five-Day Fast that I Would Recommend

In my journey to find answers for how to better cope with my multiple sclerosis, I came across a very interesting doctor whose focus was on rejuvenation. His name is Dr. Valter Longo, and I first came across his studies on TED Talks. Elsewhere, I found that he often consulted with a familiar face from our "Time-Restricted Eating" chapter, Dr. Rhonda Patrick.

Dr. Longo's research suggests that fasting is a great option for people who wish to improve their longevity. The one problem that he encountered in his research was that it's hard to get people to stick to fasting, mainly because they don't take the right incremental steps to work their way up to a longer fast period. So, he set out to create a diet that could be completed over five days, a diet which would essentially trick the body into thinking that it was in a fasting state. This fasting-mimicking diet was carried out with mice, with very promising results, as you'll see.

Dr. Longo actually started his research at UCLA studying bacteria, baker's yeast, and worms. What he found was that if these organisms were starved on only water for a specific period of time, they actually lived longer. So, in the case of bacteria, their average life extended from 36 to 84 hours. For baker's yeast, when fed they lived 15 days, whereas if they were periodically starved, they survived 45 days. And the worms, whose age capped off at around 25 days when fed, lived for 35 days when periodically starved. From this, Dr. Longo surmised that periodically starving an organism may actually lead to increased longevity. By this, he meant not only living longer with disease but living longer with a significantly decreased all-cause mortality rate.

His next study extended to mice, and what he found was that fasting also helped to conserve white blood cells while the mice were undergoing chemotherapy, an effect that we mentioned in the previous chapter. The mice in his study went through six cycles of chemotherapy, with a control group being fed and a test group fasting during the chemotherapy. The mice that were fasted during the chemotherapy were far more likely to have their white blood cell count go back to normal after the chemotherapy was over, unlike the fed mice.

After figuring out the pathways for this effect, which involve stem cell creation, Dr. Longo developed a diet that would trick the body into thinking it was fasting, which would in turn allow the activation of blood stem cells and result in regeneration and rejuvenation of the immune system. He then tested his diet out on mice, and it worked: Normally, the white blood cell count of a mouse decreases over time as the mouse ages. But when Dr. Longo put a group of older mice on his fasting-mimicking diet, their white blood cell count increased significantly to match that of younger mice.

Next, Dr. Longo placed a group of mice on a four-day fasting-mimicking diet twice a month, starting at 16 months of age, and arrived at another startling result: These mice had a much lower incidence of tumors when they reached old age, to the tune of only about 25% of the tumors seen in the control group.

So, how does this research relate to humans? Well, the process through which stem cells aid our bodies through fasting goes like this: Our bodies naturally produce stem cells; however, our access to these stem cells is normally blocked by hormones called IGF-1 and pKa. When we eliminate our intake of carbs and protein while fasting, we decrease our levels of these hormones, with the result that we our stem cells can now be accessed. Moreover, during the fasting process, we actually increase the production of stem cells, which are stored, and we decrease— through the process of autophagy—the number of auto-immune cells in our body. This means that our number of stem cells goes up while our number of immune cells goes down as we selectively get rid of the auto-immune cells through autophagy. During the process of breaking our fast (also known as refeeding), our stored stem cells are then released to create new, stronger, and better cells within the body. So, the process of breaking a fast is not the end of all fasting benefits. Refeeding ushers in healthier cells for the body to operate.

With all this in mind, Dr. Longo put together a fasting-mimicking diet for human subjects, which he had them do over the course of five days every month for three months. The results showed that after three cycles of the fasting-mimicking diet, healthy people didn't show any significant decrease in blood glucose. However, people who were pre-diabetic saw their blood glucose level return to normal on the fasting-mimicking diet.

He also tested patients at risk for cancer, measuring their rate of IGF-1, which is a marker associated with aging and cancer. After three cycles, the levels of IGF-1 for at-risk cancer patients decreased by three times that of the control group of normal patients. That is, while there was a definite decrease in IGF-1 for the normal patients, there was a *dramatic* decrease among the at-risk cancer patients.

Finally, Dr. Longo tested patients who were at risk for cardiovascular disease by measuring their C-reactive proteins, which is a risk factor for cardiovascular disease. After three cycles of his fasting-mimicking diet, there was very little change in C-reactive proteins for normal healthy people; however, there was a 150% decrease in this protein count for the at-risk group, suggesting that the fasting-mimicking diet may decrease one's risk for cardiovascular disease.

In terms of the amount of circulating stem cells in humans undergoing the fasting-mimicking diet cycles, the number of such stem cells in a normal person quadrupled after three cycles of the fasting-mimicking diet. Given that the risk for disease generally increases over time based on diet, aging, and toxins, this indication that periodic fasting or the fasting-mimicking diet can increase the number of circulating stem cells suggests a possible reduction in all age-related diseases, including but not limited to, diabetes, cancer, and Alzheimer's disease.

All of this information and research done by Dr. Longo inspired me to try the fasting-mimicking diet myself, and I would have to say that my experience was mostly positive. The only thing that prevented me from doing the fasting-mimicking diet more than twice was that I enjoyed more doing the water fast—perhaps I enjoyed the challenge of it, and it is also less expensive, as Dr. Longo's diet is essentially a package that's delivered to your home with all the food included at a cost of around $200.

So, I decided to stick with the water fast because of its practicality; however, the research that has been done by Dr. Longo can all be found through his website(prolonfast.com). I would say that if you're interested in extending your fast beyond the three-day marker, then the fasting-mimicking diet would be a much safer option than trying to do so with water alone.

Chapter Six
Spirituality and Closing

Well, that's everything that you'll need to know about short-term water fasting and why it may be your best option for fat loss, and perhaps healing from illness. I realize, though, that for some of you, the idea of fasting may seem a little bit crazy.

But is fasting really all that weird when you consider the fact that in our "hunter and gatherer" days, humans would go for days without eating? And obviously, the human race is still around. Our bodies have built-in mechanisms to handle extended periods of time without eating while still allowing us to thrive. Actually, it's really been only in the last 50 to 100 years, with the advent of modern agriculture, that we're able to eat multiple times a day and get our food conveniently at supermarkets.

Also, if you consider religions all over the world, many of them still practice fasting to this day. Jewish people fast during Yom Kippur, the Day of Atonement, and the Jewish calendar has six other fast days as well. When you consider Buddhism, all the main sects of Buddhists practice periods of fasting, usually on full moon days and other holidays. Catholics fast on Ash Wednesday and Good Friday, and they also abstain from meat on all Fridays in Lent. For Hindus, fasting is commonly practiced on new moon days and during festivals such as Shivratri, Saraswati, and Puja. Mormons, or Latter Day Saints, fast on the first day of each month. Many of these religions go back hundreds, if not thousands, of years, and maintain fasting as a focal point of their practice. And all of this is meant for spiritual cleansing, as well as rejuvenating the body. While not all religions practice water fasting per se, it's clear that there must be something basic to the idea of giving the body a chance to rest, recover, and rejuvenate.

If there's one piece of advice I can offer about fasting, it would be to take a yoga class so that you'll be better able to allow your mind to center. If not, at least allow yourself to go through a guided meditation, perhaps a five-minute one. One app that I would recommend for this purpose is called Insight Timer. Eventually, as you become better at meditating, you'll be able to go longer than five minutes. Also, as your body heals itself physically, it'll allow you to work on yourself mentally and psychologically as well. You'll find that fasting is a good opportunity to allow your thoughts to calm down and focus on whole body and mind wellness.

I wish you the best of luck with your fast and would encourage you to make sure to break your fast responsibly. I also encourage you to follow your time-restricted eating schedule strictly and to make sure that you work out two to three hours a week to get the very best results.

If you are looking for a way to be led in your exercise routines, I suggest going to www.BFFBootcamp.com where you can join any one of our virtual classes or ask about our on-demand classes. Your scale and your body fat monitor will thank you.

Best of luck to you, and God bless.

Made in United States
North Haven, CT
24 July 2022